Green Juicing For Health

Make Green Juicing Part of Your Healthy Lifestyle

RON KNESS

Contents

Disclaimer

This publication is for informational purposes only and is not intended as medical advice. Medical advice should always be obtained from a qualified medical professional for any health conditions or symptoms associated with them.

Every possible effort has been made in preparing and researching this material. We make no warranties with respect to the accuracy, applicability of its contents or any omissions.

See your healthcare professional before starting any diet or exercise program!

Introduction

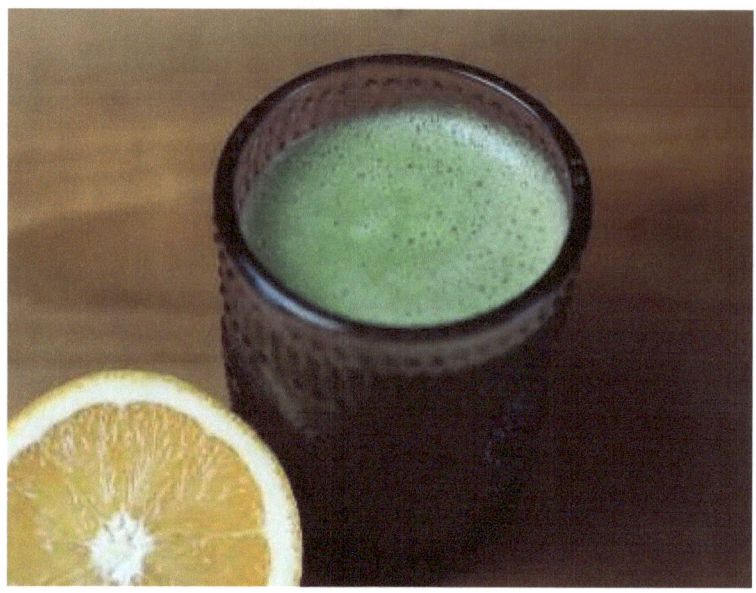

Green juicing, also known as vegetable juicing, combines a variety of leafy greens and other vegetables which are then processed through a juicer, instead of a blender.

In the fast-paced world today, time is the most precious commodity for most people, especially working professionals. In order to save time, they turn to processed foods, which include frozen meals and canned foods. They are convenient and easy to prepare.

However, eating too much processed foods could prove to be harmful for our bodies. They contain substantial amounts of saturated and trans-fats, i.e. unhealthy fats, along with sugar and salt. Prolonged intake of such foods causes people to fall sick easily. Coupled with stress in this society, it's no wonder diseases are more common and rampant among us today!

Health is wealth. As more people are becoming conscious of their health and total wellness, many have incorporated green juicing as part of their diets. It is easy to prepare and saves time. And what's more, the health benefits of green juicing are tremendous.

Health Benefits of Green Juicing

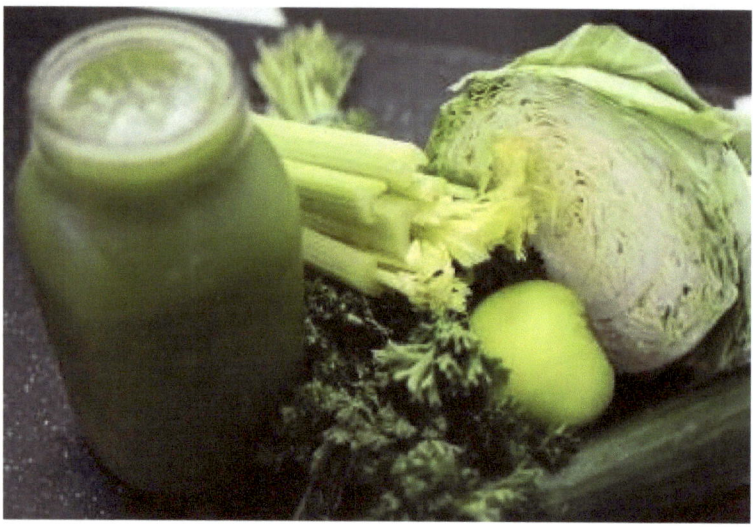

There are five basic health benefits from adding green juicing to your daily diet. They are:

- Adding Nutrients to your diet

- Beautifying your skin

- Losing weight

- Detoxing your body

- Boosting energy

Nutrients

Eating greens are good for our health and total well-being. Our bodies need to take in a certain amount of nutrients for optimal functionality.

Health authorities' recommend consuming eight servings of greens per day. Very few people actually achieve that as it means eating lots of veggies every day, which is a difficult task to accomplish. There is a limit, as far as volume or bulk, to how much food we can consume in each meal, too. Furthermore, eating too much vegetables can, in turn, cause unnecessary stress to our bodies and cause our digestive organs to be overworked.

Green juicing is a great and simple way to get large amounts of veggies into our system, without overworking our organs. We can get in the recommended one day's worth of nutrients from fresh greens all in just one glass. When we drink vegetable juice, minerals, vitamins, and enzymes are absorbed directly into our system. As a result, these nutrients do not have to be further broken down, and thus cause our organs to be overworked.

Fresh vegetables contain insoluble fibers which makes absorbing certain nutrients into our bodies difficult. Instead of eating and chewing on fresh produce, green juicing allows our bodies to absorb these nutrients better.

For those with digestion problems, drinking vegetable juice is a great way for the body to absorb lots of nutrients from vegetables which may otherwise be difficult if they were to eat fresh produces. This is made possible as the fiber, which may cause digestion problems, is separated from the juice.

Beautiful Skin

Drinking freshly made vegetable juices everyday can have an excellent effect on our skin's texture and tone. Recent studies have shown that people with skin woes such as skin blemishes, acne, blackheads, or redness who increased their consumption of fresh vegetables have found that their skin texture has become clearer and smoother. In fact, their skin glows according to the research.

The state of our skin reflects the state of our inner health. Our skin is the main way that our bodies detoxify. When we eat deep-fried and processed foods, our bodies will try to get rid of the harmful substances known as toxins. If we do not take enough vegetables to purge these toxins out through our system, the toxins will be pushed out through the skin and cause acne, blemishes and other skin disorders.

While we treat our skin disorders with external facial applications which helps to a certain extent, we should also treat these disorders from the inside-out.

Great skin is created from the inside. In order to keep it strong, supple, and clear, it will need a constant stream of all-natural nutrients, such as minerals, anti-oxidants, vitamins, and enzymes that can be highly absorbed. Drinking green juices will provide the needed nutrients for healthy skin.

Eating raw and fresh foods helps clears up our skin. Most vegetables are high in anti-oxidants which protect our skin from free radicals. It also helps speed up the repair of damaged cells and skin regeneration which gives us glowing skin.

It helps to reduce any signs of premature aging too!

Lose Weight

When drinking a glass of fresh green juice, we are loading our bodies with minerals contained in these vegetables that help to detoxify our bodies. These nutrients allow us to heal, minimize the risk of sicknesses, and thus stay healthy. As a result, it reduces our cravings for processed foods and sweets that, most often than not, add on extra pounds to our bodies.

When we drink vegetable juices, we are feeding what our bodies actually need. And because our bodies get what is needed, it suppresses our appetite and keeps us full. Our bodies will not send signals to our brains that make us crave for certain foods, especially bad foods that put extra pounds on us, that has certain vitamins or minerals we are lacking. Our stomachs won't get hunger pangs that will make us look for more food.

Contrary to popular belief that green juices taste yucky, it actually tastes great. You can vary the juice concoction to make it even more flavorful and tasty by adding mint or ginger. You can even add lemon too. You'll surely enjoy the juice so much that you'll choose to make vegetable juice over eating unhealthy snacks when you do get those hunger pangs.

With lesser food intake and more nutrition from drinking green juices, it will surely cause us to lose those extra pounds.

Body Detox

The environment that we live in today is full of pollutants and harmful particles in the air. Unknowingly, we absorb these harmful substances into our bodies, and thus cause damages to our bodies. Coupled with the unhealthy foods, i.e. processed foods, that we eat, it's no wonder our bodies are so full of toxins that they need to be cleared out.

Digestion problems, bad skin, headaches, brittle hair and nails, body pains and aches are indications of toxins in our bodies. When toxins are not eliminated properly, it will cause these problems to surface. If you're struggling with any of these problems, it's time for a body cleanse.

Body detoxification, or body cleansing, is a process of clearing our body of toxins. It is about nourishing and cleaning our bodies from the inside out. In a body detox, our colons and kidneys are cleansed as these organs are responsible for removing toxins from our bodies. Cleansing our bodies protects us from diseases and keeps us in optimum health.

Green juicing is a great way to detox our bodies. It not only refuels our bodies with healthy nutrients that our bodies need, it also helps to stimulate the liver to eliminate the toxins out of our bodies. Furthermore, it improves blood circulation too.

Drinking green juices helps our digestive systems to function properly. Toxins and unwanted wastes that has accumulated will move through our digestive systems quickly, making us feel much healthier.

Energy Booster

Coffee is known as an energy booster and because of it, most people turn to coffee when they want that extra kick. A cup of coffee cannot last you through the day, however. Added sugars in coffee can cause a surge in energy, and a crash later on. It can give you a sudden boost after one cup, but your energy will wear out leaving you to consume your next cup of coffee three to four hours later. More often than not, you'll have to consume three to four cups a day for that boost in energy you're looking for.

While drinking coffee has its advantages, such as helping you lose weight, staying alert and focusing, reducing cancer risks, and minimizing the risks of stroke, it has its own set of disadvantages. In the extreme, an overdose of caffeine can actually kill you. In large quantities, coffee is toxic which can cause sicknesses, headaches, restlessness and insomnia.

Instead of reaching for your caffeinated drink, why not drink green juice in place of coffee? It has all the benefits that coffee has, plus more! It is more rejuvenating, and is the perfect wake-up drink and a refresher in the afternoons.

The nutrients in the vegetables is food for every cell in our bodies. The green pigment, also known as chlorophyll, helps in blood circulation, thereby increasing brain function and boost energy.

Green Juicing Vs Green Smoothies

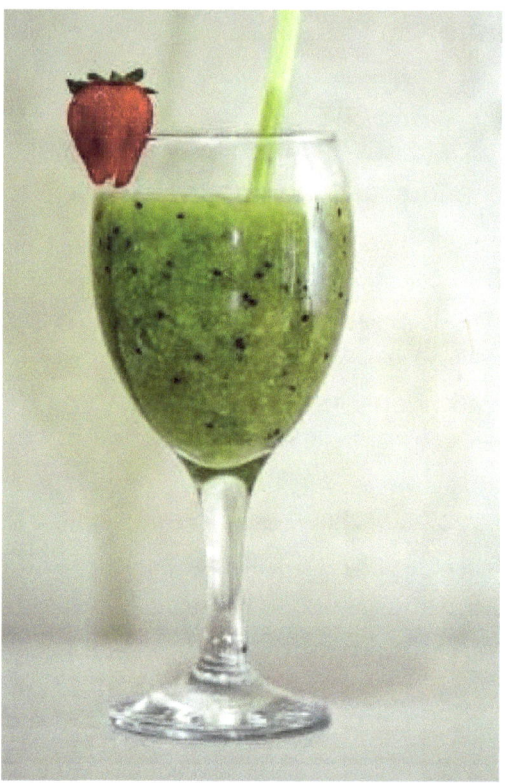

Green vegetables are the most healing and healthy food on earth. They contain loads of vitamins and nutrients that our bodies need. They are alkaline and contain cancer-fighting agents to help fight against cancer.

To ensure that we get optimal nutrition, we'll need to consume at least 0.5 lbs of fresh greens every day. It won't be possible with normal consumption of whole fresh vegetables. Furthermore, there is a limit as to how much we can eat, and most of these greens aren't tasty when eaten raw. This is when blending and juicing greens come into play.

Both blending and juicing are perfect for incorporating lots of fresh produce into our diets. They are great ways to consume far more than what we could otherwise eat. For those vegetables we hate eating, we can turn them into tasty treats by incorporating and mixing them up with other vegetables and fruits by blending or juicing.

Most people are confused about the differences between the two, and they believe that they are juicing when they are actually blending. There is, however, one main difference, and that is in the pulp.

Whether we choose to juice or blend, we are infusing our bodies with nutrient-packed drinks. Regularly drinking either one or both will curb our appetites and reduce our cravings for processed foods and sugar. We are providing our cells with what they need and, in return, our bodies no longer crave for unhealthy foods. It also helps our bodies absorb the nutrients more quickly and easily because the foods are pre-digested in juicing or blending.

Green Juicing

In green juicing, a juicer is used to extract the juice, including water and nutrients, and leaving the pulp, the insoluble fiber, behind. When juicing, the juice is separated from the pulp, which is then discarded.

Fiber is beneficial to us as it keeps our digestive systems healthy and helps to slow down sugar absorption into our bodies. However good for us, the fact is that fiber also prevents nutrients from being absorbed into our bodies. Furthermore, some nutrients remain in the pulp that our bodies will not get.

When the pulp is separated from the juice, our bodies are able to absorb all the nutrients, giving us a boost in energy instantly. In juicing, the nutrients are readily available to be absorbed because our bodies do not have to break down the components of the food. Seventy percent of the nutrients goes right into the glass when we juice.

For those fresh greens we don't usually eat, like beets or kale, green juicing allows us to experiment with them. These vegetables we may not like are usually packed full of nutrients and vitamins we may not get in other vegetables.

One thing to take note is that we can't replace a meal with green juicing, as it's not a main source of protein. Fibers and proteins are what's needed to keep us full. Without these two nutrients, it will be hard for us not to feel hungry.

However, If you're looking to boost your fresh produce intake, then green juicing is the way to go!

Green Smoothie

Blenders are used to make smoothies. Green smoothie involves blending the whole produce including its pulp into smoothie. Nothing is removed or separated. The pulp is not removed when blending. The final produce is thicker than juicing, as the pulp and fiber is in it.

Drinking green smoothies allows you to greatly increase the vegetables intake per day. It is a 'fast food' for busy people who have no time to cook. It's a great meal replacement, whereas juicing is not.

If you're looking for a quick nutrients-packed snack or meal that will keep your hunger pangs at bay, then go for green smoothies.

Pros and Cons

Now that we know the differences between green juicing and green smoothie, let's take a look at the pros and cons of each method.

Green Juicing Pros

- More vegetable servings per glass - Pulp is removed when you juice. Because of that, more vegetable juice will be able to fit into the glass as compared to smoothie.

- Gives you instant rush of energy - Juicing produces a higher concentration of vegetables and nutrients in one glass than smoothie. Our bodies do not need to do the hard work of digesting the veggies because juicing produces pre-digested veggies that enables our bodies to absorb the nutrients much quicker.

- Makes digesting nutrients easier - Juicing draws water and nutrients out from vegetables, leaving behind the pulps and fibers. Unlike smoothie, these nutrients go straight into our body systems without having to use our energy to digest all the fibers.

- Enzymes not destroyed - Unlike blending, juicers do not have high-speed blades that, when run, causes the juices to be slightly heated.

And this can kill off the enzymes that are beneficial to us.

Green Juicing Cons

- *Fiber content -* The recommended daily fiber intake is at least 25g. The average an American gets currently is only 15g a day. Because juicing removes the fiber from the vegetables we juice, we'll need to get enough fiber intake from other sources of fruits and vegetables.

- Difficult to clean juicers - Cleaning juicers is a bit cumbersome, as juicers consist of more parts than in blenders. It also takes a longer time to clean too.

- Need to buy more vegetables - Green juicing requires more vegetables per serving than blending. Therefore, we need to buy more vegetables, which will cost more.

- More space required in refrigerator - Because more vegetables are required for green juicing, we would need more space to store them too.

Green Smoothie Pros

- Fiber keeps us full longer - When blending, the fiber is not removed from the vegetable, and is consumed together with the veggies. Fiber fills up the space in our stomachs and keep us full longer. This prevents us from getting hungry and eating unnecessary.

- Minimal costs - Less vegetables are required, and therefore cost less than juicing. Furthermore, we do not need special equipment to make green smoothies. Most households would have already own a blender in their home.

- Add a little flavor - If you or your kids don't like the tastes of vegetables, you can throw in fruits, milk, nuts, etc. into the blender to make it more flavorful. You and your kids will love it!

Green Smoothie Cons

- Less nutrients per serving - As the fiber stays in smoothies, we'll need to drink lots of smoothies to get the same amount of nutrients, minerals and vitamins we get from drinking one glass of juice.

- Some vegetables not suitable for blending - Some vegetables, especially root vegetables, like sweet potatoes, beets and carrots are not suitable for blending. They don't taste good, and come off as bitter. They're more suitable for juicing.

How to Green Juice When You Dislike the Tastes of Vegetable Juice

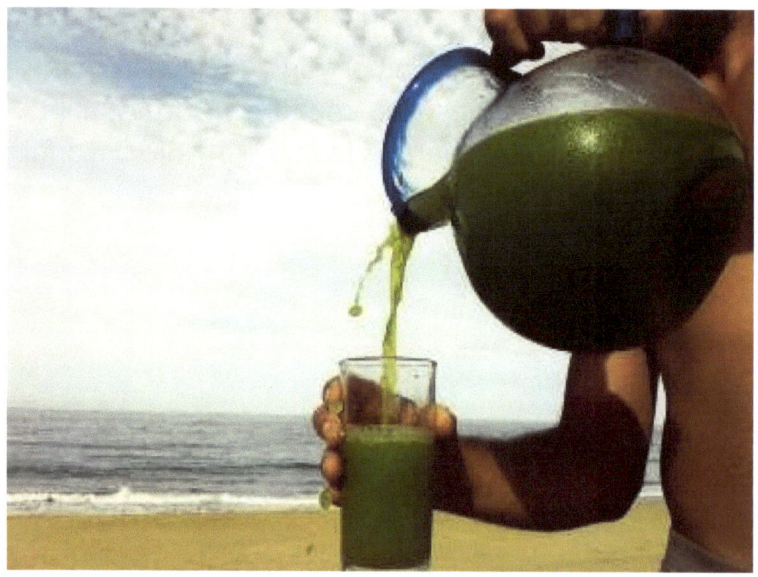

A recent survey found around 30% of the people living in the States fear green juices. The lack of fondness towards these drinks may come out as a surprise for most people, considering their unmatched health benefits. Well, it's not actually the color, or the appearance that they find unattractive; it's only that bitter taste.

People who decide to start green juicing routines often choose to step out of it soon, and it's because of the same reason mentioned above; the flavor. Celery, most certainly, would never taste like the fruity tart smoothies that they may be used to. It's vital to keep in mind while signing up for green juicing that you're not in it for the taste, but you're looking for physical wellness.

For someone who appreciates it, there's also a good side to a glass full of juiced up vegetables. You'll most definitely find a lot to feel good about as you drink these green juices, knowing it's best for your body.

"I love to create this green juice shake made from kale, spinach, cucumber and wheatgrass. The nutrients in the juice help me recover after a tough workout. The Kale Banana Smoothie at LYFE Kitchen is very similar to my recipe and is fantastic." – Troy Polamalu.

If someone as strong as Troy Polamalu loves to indulge in green juicing recipes, you'd know there's something to them that's worth all the bitter trouble.

What Makes People Continue Green Juicing?

Reminding yourself of the countless advantages of green juices is the major key to keep away the hatred you may have for them. If you're looking to make progress in this practice of green juicing, you'll have to learn to overlook the only flaw there is to it; occasional bitterness.

Green juices tend to alkalize our bodies very effectively, and the benefits of a properly alkalized body are numerous. A few such health pros worth mentioning are:

- A much more elastic and youthful feel over the skin.
- Deeper and more effective sleep cycles.
- Increased physical energy.
- Prevention against flu, cold, and migraines.
- A better level of concentration and mental alertness.
- Improved digestion.
- A naturally occurring sense of calm.
- Lesser chances for arthritis and osteoporosis to occur.

Besides the alkalizing properties of green juices, it's worth mentioning that they are also rich in anti-oxidants. Anti-oxidants have been found to contain various healthful properties, including prevention against a lethal disease; cancer. Isn't that all worth a chug of slight bitterness every day? In fact, people have reviewed a few recipes as highly likeable too, as they progress into the world of green juicing.

How to NOT Hate Green Juicing
Definitely, there are ways you can adopt that will hugely reduce the chances of you deciding that you've had enough, and ultimately quitting. It is not going to be an easy practice as a starter, but with the right tips and techniques, you'll surely have a better shot at keeping it up. If you don't like vegetable juice and still wish to start a green juicing habit, given below are the tips you will need.

Keep the routine going:
After attaining a clear realization of the fact that you want these green drinks to be a part of your life, the next step is to convince your taste buds to make a few compromises. Good news is that there are ways to potentially change what we like, in terms of taste. Repeat exposure has been found to be the most effective way to acclimate our taste buds. This means, that if you stick with the bitterness for long enough, you may actually start fancying it.

Quit comparing:
Green juices would surely taste different from what you'd normally like to drink. However, savoring a new taste, and accepting it for whatever it is, is an experience in itself.

Comparing them with a soda or a cold drink would only cause one to lose what's best about the journey of green juicing; a unique flavor of something that enters your body for your own good. For instance, *Mountain Dew* could be fun to sip, but it certainly won't prevent cancer.

Go For Some Other Color:
Yes, green juicing could involve shades other than green too. It's all about juicing up vegetables, basically. Carrots will add an orange color to your juices, while beets tend to give your drinks a gorgeous shade of magenta. Turmeric roots can be used to shift the whole color scheme into a tint of yellow. In a few cases, people have found the changed coloration of the juices helpful in taking these drinks down.

Sweeten It Up, but Not with Sugar:
Making your green juices a bit more flavorful with a few slices of fruit won't oppose the positive effects of vegetables. Fruits have their own benefits too, and the only benefit we're mainly concerned about when it comes to their role in green juicing, is that they are sweet. Putting in a few pear slices, or some chunks of pineapple or Kiwi in the juicer, could make the drink much more enjoyable. It's a great tip for the beginners!

Bitter is the Culprit:
As a starter who doesn't like vegetable juice, it would be advisable for you to minimize the bitterness in your green juice recipes. Pairing up bitter vegetables with mellower ones, such as Celery with Kale, could turn out to be much less unlikeable. The combinations you go for play a big role in how much you're going to dislike this habit in the start.

Cucumber:
Adding a cucumber in almost all the green juicing recipes wouldn't be a bad idea in the start. Cucumber tends to balance out bitterness in most cases, which will prove to be very helpful.

It technically is a fruit itself, but it's green, so it counts.

Likeable Green Juicing Recipes for Beginners

Now that we've learned the tips you needed to know before stepping into the world of green juicing, it's time to go over a few specific drinks that you'll find a lot easier to chug as a beginner. The green juices mentioned below are mainly meant for people who've just started this practice, and quite understandably, do not like the bitter taste of Kale and Broccoli.

The following recipes look to add suitable fruits into the blend, while keeping the purpose of green juicing alive. Experts suggest that 80% of these green drinks should be produced only by vegetables. Keeping this number in mind, here are the drinks that will suit you best!

Perfectly Sweet Romaine - Ingredients:

- Romaine Lettuce
- Carrots
- Apple

The most attractive thing about this recipe, besides the palatable sweet flavor, is that the aforementioned items are one of the cheapest to be found at the store. The Romaine will definitely add that healthy green color to your drink, while hardly changing the flavor.

Apple & Kale – Ingredients:

- Apple
- Kale
- Lemon

These two, being the opposite to each other in terms of flavor, bring out the best in each other when accompanied by some lemon juice. Sure, Kale comes with bitterness, but the other two ingredients work swimmingly to stabilize it. This is as healthy as it gets for something that tastes as good as an extra sour apple juice.

Rise and Shine – Ingredients:

- Cucumber
- Celery
- Cinnamon
- Apple
- Ginger

This drink, as the name suggests, helps in making your mornings a lot fresher by being filled with the hydration that celery and cucumber provide. Apple and cinnamon carve a desirable combo, making this healthy drink a delight for the beginners.

Verdant Intermediate – Ingredients:

- Wheatgrass
- Kale/Spinach
- Cucumber
- Celery

Now these ingredients must sound like a complete flavor disaster, but rest assured, the taste isn't too bland with this one. This recipe is the healthiest of the ones mentioned here, but at the same time, it's mild. Feel free to squeeze in a lemon in it if you feel like you're not ready for this one yet.

Spring Cooler – Ingredients:

- Mint
- Cucumber
- Apple
- Ginger Root

The one ingredient which makes this green juice stand out is mint. It does not get more refreshing than this. The apple works to sweeten the blend up for your taste buds, while the cucumber and ginger root are the ones you'll benefit the most from.

Melon Carrot Juice – Ingredients:

- Carrot
- Orange
- Melon

This one's a personal favorite. The bright orange coloration of this drink lightens up the whole green juicing routine. The orange & carrot combo is a pretty common one, and these two ingredients are something you'll be blending together a lot as you progress further as a green juicer. Here, melon plays a vital role in making this blend naturally sweet, brighter, and a delightful breakfast-friendly item.

Common Green Juicing Mistakes

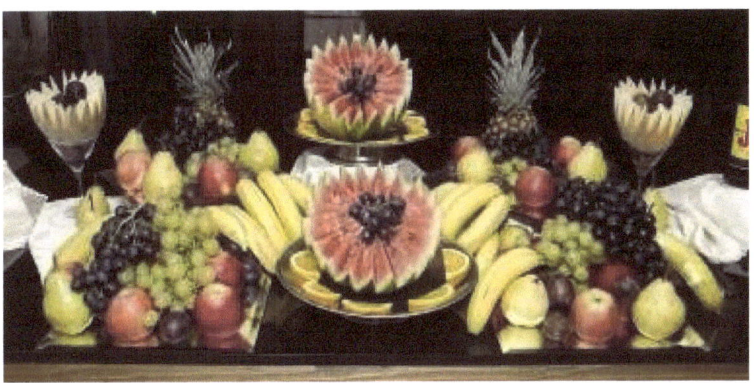

Juicing, as simple as it may sound, could prove to be a complicated practice to maintain if it's started without acquiring sufficient knowledge about it. It brings a lot of pitfalls with it that are to be avoided once a person starts following these routines.

Many consider this practice to be more of a 'freestyle' fitness habit, which is true, in most cases. Sure, green juicing followers could throw in veggies of their choice to craft a recipe of their own, and that's completely fine. However, numerous problems may arise unknowingly due to the lack of knowledge.

Whether it's an excess of fruit slices in the vegetable juice, or letting the juice sit for too long; all these mistakes are commonly made due to the absence of awareness. Mentioned below are various mistakes that are seen to be commonly made by green juicing practitioners.

Too Bitter! More Fruit!

This mistake could be the most common one that beginner juicers make. They'll throw in kale, broccoli, celery, spinach in the juicer all at the same time, and wonder why it ends up tasting undrinkable. To make it 'drinkable', they tend to add unacceptable amounts of sweetening fruits and ultimately even the bitterness out.

Sugar is to be generally avoided, and the whole concept of juicing centers on that precaution. Green juicing is meant to revamp your body's nutrition, and adding too many sugary fruits would be the exact opposite of that.

There's always going to be bitterness in green beverages, be it just a hint of it or something that makes it an unpalatable blend. All you can do is make it milder by adding some lemon juice or throwing **a few** slices of apple or some other naturally sweeter fruit.

Similar Timings Do NOT Apply to Everybody:

If you're a beginner and don't know when to consume your juices, then imitating a fitness trainer without proper consultation wouldn't be the best idea for you. The reason behind this is that each human body has a different metabolism, and that's what the suitability of timings depends upon the most.

Keeping a few general things in mind, you'll know when to drink up a glass. According to experts, the best time to consume juices is early morning, before breakfast.

The logic behind this seems pretty clear: the body would be able to soak up the nutrients entirely as it won't have to digest something you had swallowed prior to the juice.

Besides early mornings, green juices are found to be great post workout drinks as well. After some intense exercises at the gym, the body's glucose levels are likely to be at their lowest, and that's when the sugary sweets in your juices won't be converted into fat. The sugar from the fruits will be used up to maintain the glucose levels that went down during your gym session. This allows you to enjoy a tastier juice without having to pay the price for it.

Forgetting the Golden Rule of Proportion

It is known to almost every juicer who's somewhat experienced that all the green juicing recipes must have at least 80% of pure veggies and only 20% of fruits may be added as flavoring.

This rule is directly linked to the mistake mentioned first. As long as the 80/20 rule is followed, it's all okay to be as innovative as you'd like with your recipes. If your fruit quantity exceeds from what is allowed by this rule, you'll have started to make your green juice ineffective in terms of health beneficiary.

Keeping the Juice Waiting When It Is Ready:

Vegetable juices tend to lose their most important advantages if they're left to wait even when they're ready to be drunk.

Juices, when kept outside their production machines, will be exposed to oxygen and heat; these two are the biggest destroyers of vital minerals and vitamins.

Juices made with centrifugal machines (having larger number of rotations per minute), have a much higher rate of losing these important resources when exposed to oxygen and heat.

Due to these reasons, it is highly recommended to consume your green juices as soon as they're ready.

However, if they were made using a masticating juicer, then they can be comfortably stored in a refrigerator for 2-3 days. Personally, this choice too seems much of a risk, and nothing beats the natural freshness of a vegetable juice.

Not Considering Masticating Juicers:

It's always recommended by experts to use a masticating juicer over a centrifugal one. Cold processed drinks are almost a must in this practice, and masticating machines ensure the production of much lesser heat in the procedure of blending the vegetables. Due to its low RPM (Rotations per Minute) value, the vegetables have a lower chance of losing their vital benefits.

A masticating juicer may not be as affordable as the other kind is, but it sure is something that you should consider saving up for.

It's a good idea to opt for an Omega branded juicer for a start, as they produce these juicers at relatively lower rates with almost the same advantages. I've included a review of an Omega model toward the end of this book.

Bottom's up! No Time to Taste, No Time to Waste:

Have you been drinking it all in one big gulp, in less than 30 seconds? That's a move that you should never opt for with green juices. People not wanting to taste the bitter fury for a long time often go for this technique.

As much as you'd hate your green juices in the start, experienced practitioners actually view them as something enjoyable. Where's the fun in chugging it all down your throat in a matter of seconds? If it takes so much time to prepare and clean up after that, shouldn't you be savoring the taste for a bit longer than that?

Apart from that, this move is inadvisable from a health perspective as well. Digestion doesn't only happen inside your stomach, but it starts from your mouth. Chew your juice, and keep your sips in your mouth for a few seconds to appreciate the green awesomeness! Doing this will help the juice to mix with your saliva before being swallowed, enhancing the health benefits in some cases.

Same Juices Every Day

Experts preach people must not only indulge in green juicing because of its healthful effects, but the whole process should be enjoyed as it is. The chances of green juicing being 'enjoyed' are negligible if the recipes aren't switched up every morning.

Try out a variety of different combinations of fruits and vegetables to discover the one you'd think is best. Majorly, the fun of green juicing lies in the diversity and the wide range of mishmashes.

Come up with a creative and fulfilling schedule every week. This way, your body gets to have different kinds of nutrition, which helps in fighting different kinds of problems each morning.

Thinking Juices Can Replace Solid Foods... For Good!

As people get more and more into green juicing, their enthusiasm for the practice may push them to the phase where they start thinking they don't need solid food anymore. This is a completely wrong ideology to even consider adopting.

A juice cleanse may work effectively for a matter of a couple days, but in the long run, you should only consume vegetable juices as a supplement to use along with foods.

Comparing Fresh Green Juices with Bottled Products:

You might have heard people saying stuff like "Oh, I can just walk to the supermarket and buy some for myself" to regular green juicing practitioners. This comparison is completely baseless, as it's literally like comparing plain white sugar to a majestic blend of vitamins, minerals, and cancer preventing anti-oxidants.

Most of these branded shelved juices in the supermarket are basically dead inside, and have no valuable resources that your body could potentially benefit from. A large number of these products are heated intentionally to kill all the bacteria, consequently killing the much needed vitamins and minerals too. All there is to them left is sugar, and that's what we're trying to dodge.

Veggie Cocktail – Let's Give that a Try:

That's actually a bad idea. While you should be encouraged to throw in multiple ingredients and find what mixture you love, 5 ingredients should be considered the limit.

People have tried to blend together ten different vegetables and fruits; the same people then wonder what made their drink taste like trash. It's best to start with two or three different things, while carefully adding more once you figure out what's missing. It's the most enjoyable that way.

You should be able to make out what flavor is coming from which ingredient when you are savoring the taste of the mixture in the end; that's the key.

Getting Farther Away from Plain Water:

Interestingly, most vegetables consist of 50%-60% water themselves. However, nothing will hydrate your system as effectively as pure water itself. A lot of problems arise due to the lack of water in the body, and you must realize how important it is to keep yourself properly hydrated while going for any of these diet routines.

Drinking two to three liters of water per day will ensure proper hydration for your bodies. People, who exercise regularly and/or intensively, would need to drink a lot more than that.

Green Juicing Side Effects

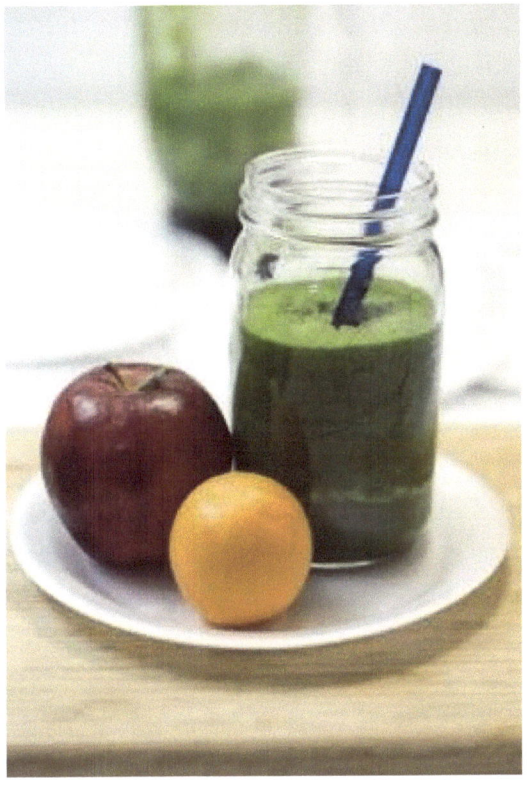

Whenever you make changes to your normal routine - especially when it comes to eating - there are bound to be some adjustments that your body will experience. With green juicing, there are some side effects that you'll want to be aware of.

These side effects are mild and do pass rather quickly. But there are ways to handle them and even prevent them in some cases, so awareness is key in making your green juicing experience a positive one.

Low Calorie Juicing Side Effects

If you want to find a way to get healthier, leaner and stave off potential health issues, then green juicing is one of the best ways to do that. When you first get started, you'll notice a difference in the way that you feel.

You will have more energy from all of the nutrients. On the flip side though, since most people are usually consuming far more calories than they realize before a juicing cleanse, when they switch to juicing, they usually find that they experience an increase in hunger pangs.

This will subside as the stomach adjusts to this new, healthier way of eating. You simply have to wait it out. What you can also do is if you find that the hunger pangs are too annoying to deal with, is add a few more calories to your diet and lower them slowly instead of all at once.

This allows your body time to get used to the change rather than going cold turkey. While you will experience an upswing in energy, it's also fairly common to experience fatigue for some people.

The reason this happens is because most people are accustomed to consuming meals that contain a large volume of carbohydrates. Carbohydrates, especially slow acting ones, remain in the body longer and take longer to digest.

Carbs keep your glucose level up. Without the same high level of carbs, your glucose level will lower and level out. So you'll experience a bit of exhaustion. This will go away once your body goes through the adjustment period and then your energy levels surge higher than before.

Another common side effect of low calorie juicing is mood changes. Hunger is a common cause of irritability. Because you'll be eating less, it will be easier to become irritated.

This is something that is fleeting and will also go away. The majority of people who start a low calorie juicing lifestyle do it after having been accustomed to eating a certain type of food on a regular basis.

So when you change that - especially if you do it suddenly - it can throw your digestive system out of whack. You might go through periods where you need to have frequent bowel movements or you might experience the opposite - constipation.

Most people, however, will deal with more frequency. If you give your body time to accustom, your bathroom habits will stabilize.

You may also notice a difference in your glucose readings if you're diabetic. Juicing can cause elevated readings and you might feel fatigue, thirsty and tired.

If that happens, you'll simply need to adjust the amount of fruit (sugar) you have in your concoctions. For people who choose to use the low calorie green juicing as a means of detoxing, they'll experience similar side effects.

But they may also start to have headaches or to experience dizziness. This is completely normal as well. It's caused by lowering the amount of calories that you're used to eating.

If you're someone who was big on drinking caffeine and you go off of it for the detox, then withdrawing from the caffeine can cause both headaches and irritability.

All of these symptoms will pass within 48 hours.

Low Fiber Side Effects with Green Juicing

Green juicing is a great way to get plenty of nutrients in your daily diet. Most people actually get the daily recommended amount of fiber when they have an eating plan that includes juicing.

However, if you're not careful and aren't paying attention, then you can accidentally leave a good portion of the pulp in your juicer. When that happens, the beverages that you're creating aren't getting the right amount of fiber content - which means you're not getting it, either.

That can equal a diet that's too low in fiber. A diet that doesn't contain enough fiber can throw off your normal digestive routine. When that happens, you'll experience side effects that can make you uncomfortable.

One of these side effects is bloating. With bloating, you can feel pain in your abdomen. You can also experience gas and burping as a result of this bloating, caused by low fiber.

Not having enough fiber can cause you to have constipation and when that happens, you'll struggle to go the bathroom or end up producing stools that are hard to pass. While low fiber can definitely be a problem when green juicing, it does have a simple remedy to fixing all of the side effects associated with it.

You just need to make sure that you get all the pulp out of your juicer when you're making your beverages. Sometimes, people don't get enough fiber when green juicing because they're not aware of how to use the fiber dense foods when creating the drinks.

This is also an easy problem to resolve. You just need to make sure that you know which foods offer you the amount of fiber that you need. These will be foods such as apples, broccoli, carrots and more.

It's easier to get the fiber you need when you're able to follow recipes that tell you the fiber content. These recipes are found in books that contain recipes dedicated to green juicing.

Loss of Muscle Mass on a Green Juicing Diet

The beneficial effects of green juicing are well known. You can feel better, look better, have more energy, gain a boost in your immune system and lose weight - which in turn contributes to better long term health.

However, one of the side effects of being on a green juicing diet is that you might experience a loss of muscle mass if you're not careful. It's true that the foods you'll consume in juicing are excellent resources for your body, but you need essential amino acids in order to give your muscles what they need to thrive.

If you don't, then what happens is that your body will begin to take the protein from areas of your body - specifically your muscles.

This is known as muscle wasting, because without the proper amount of protein, muscles just can't function the way they're supposed to.

The side effects of a lack of protein are pretty obvious. You'll start to experience more soreness in your muscles, even if you're not being overly active. You'll also notice that your muscles feel weaker than they used to - as if they've given up some of their strength (and that's because they have).

The lack of protein robs your muscles of their strength. You'll begin to lose the muscle mass and you'll discover that your muscles just don't work the way they were once able to.

This loss of muscle mass that occurs when someone is on a green juicing diet isn't something that has to happen. When it happens, it's usually because the person on the diet isn't paying enough attention to their body's nutritional demands.

You must have protein - even on a green juicing diet. Thankfully, making sure you get the protein that you need on this diet is a quick and easy fix. You just have to make sure that you're using ingredients that contain the protein that you need.

This is why you need a guide or some kind of recipe book or instructional help to teach you how to keep the protein during a green juicing diet. What you can do to fix it right now is you can add certain ingredients to your beverages.

You can add chia seeds for one. These contain around 4 grams of protein. Another protein you can add is ground flax seeds. These contain around 5 grams of protein.

If you already haven't been getting enough protein and you're already feeling some of the side effects, then add ingredients with a higher protein count such as hemp seeds, which contain about 10 grams of protein.

You can also use protein powder as long as you choose the kind that doesn't contain any artificial flavorings, color or sugars. Simply add a scoop of protein to the blender or to the juiced concoction and you'll prevent deterioration of your muscles and strength.

Energy Boost By Weeding Out Food Allergies

Green juicing can make you feel great. The first couple of days will be an adjustment period for you. You'll be eating a different way and then dealing with the side effects that will happen as a result of that.

You'll discover that you have a lot of energy and you won't feel bogged down or bloated with food. An added benefit with green juicing that's closely linked to how you feel and how much energy you have is found in food allergies.

Food allergies are fairly common, but there are many people who aren't even aware that they have them. They just know that they don't feel the best that they could feel. When you're green juicing or going through a cleanse, you're cutting out the foods that can be causing you to have allergies that you know about - and in some cases, don't know about.

Some of the more common allergies are found in dairy, nuts, and wheat - though this is just the tip of the iceberg when it comes to allergies.

Many foods are cross developed, so you may think you're eating something that's free of everything you have an allergy to - when you're actually consuming trace amounts of it.

When you cut out the things that trigger your allergies, something amazing takes place within your body. You can end up not having the abdominal issues that you've dealt with for ages.

You can stop feeling bloated, not have issues with gas or gas pains, and you can stop feeling like you're sick to your stomach. When you get away from foods that trigger your allergies, you'll notice an improvement in symptoms that are connected to the foods that you eat.

You can diminish or end headaches that you may have struggled with. Your body can stop feeling like you're so fatigued or achy. If you go on a green juice diet or a detox cleanse and you notice that you feel better by the second day, that can be a good sign that you could have been dealing with a food allergy and may not have realized it.

Being on the green juice diet or detoxing can help you narrow down the food that's the cause of making you feel less than your best. You can use this for what it is - an opportunity to slowly add back one food at a time.

When you add that food back, if your symptoms rear up, then you'll be able to identify what it is that's caused you to feel bad or have a reaction. Understand that sometimes, when you go on a green juicing diet or a detox, cutting out certain foods can be triggers in themselves.

Since caffeine is a stimulant, cutting that out can actually cause headaches to develop. It can also cause irritability and mood swings when cutting it out cold turkey. It's a firm sign that your body was being artificially propped up to keep you going throughout the day.

Detox Symptoms That Affect Hormones and Senses

Whenever you're doing a detox, you can expect that you're going to experience some symptoms as your body adjusts. Some of these symptoms are going to play a hand in how your hormones and senses function.

This is a natural reaction and your body will adapt quickly. As toxins leave your body, you might actually feel worse when you begin the cleanse, but this doesn't last long. You might feel like you're coming down with something and get headaches.

You might experience fatigue, dizziness and bowel changes. Again, all of this is perfectly normal and these symptoms don't last through the entire cleanse. You're not only ridding your body of the things that aren't that healthy for you, but you're also putting your body through a food change and it will give off symptoms as it does that.

During the first couple of days of a detox, you're not going to feel your best. But if you can make it over the hurdle and get through those days, then you'll feel amazing. For women, one of the ways that detoxing affects the hormones is through menstrual cycle alterations.

Some women won't experience any changes in this area, while others might have a missed period or additional period as the body adjusts. Once it does, however, the cycle will resume its regular routine.

Detoxing can also decrease the feelings and symptoms associated with PMS. The changes in your hormones that occur with detoxing can sometimes show up on your skin.

Some people will see changes such as a sudden increase or outbreak of acne or red or blotchy areas on the skin. This is normal and is caused by the toxins leaving the body as well as the ingredients you may be using in the cleanse.

This side effect will right itself within a day or two of the cleanse. A detox can affect your senses by causing you to taste or smell things that you no longer take part in - such as drinking alcohol or smoking.

Your body may call up these phantom tastes and smells as a result of the body getting rid of the toxins associated with the habit. This won't last long and your sense of taste and smell will return to normal.

Green juicing, like many other health and weight loss journeys, is an adjustment period for your body and mind. While you may have to deal with a few minor discomforts, they are far outweighed by the tremendous energy and health benefits you'll experience if you get over the 48-hour hurdle.

How to Get the Most Out of Green Juicing

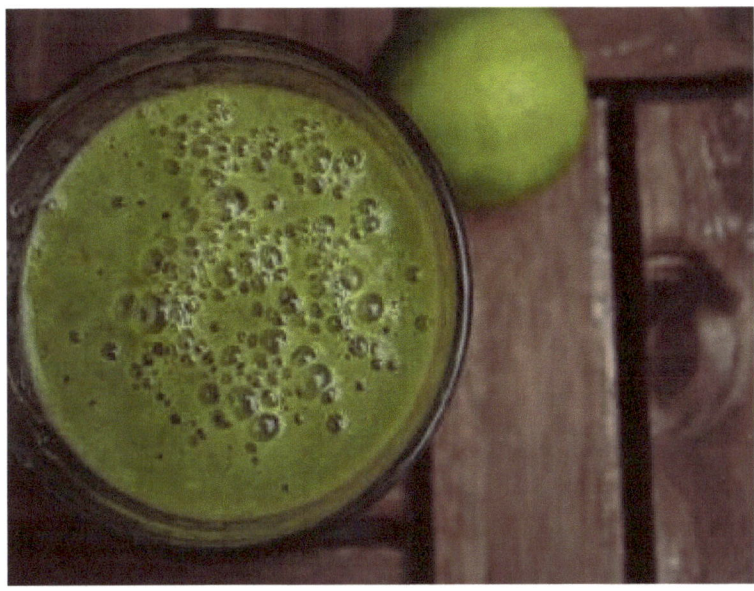

Green juicing comes with its complexities, and only a small error in your everyday juicing regularities could potentially make you lose what's best about them, in the long run. As we've gotten to know earlier, if your centrifugally blended green juice waits for you for hours out in the open, there's high chance you've killed the most vital nutrients and vitamins in it. These types of errors are what we need to look out for in this journey.

Prevention from the loss of valuable minerals is one thing, but could you essentially enhance their healthful effects with some more tips? Could you actually learn to like these drinks a bit more as you progress through your days? The answer is, yes!

Given below are the basic do's and don'ts of green juicing that will help you make the most out of your juicing routines.

Keeping it Clean:

It's extremely important that your vegetables get thoroughly uncontaminated and washed before they are thrown into the juicer. Though it could be challenging to fully clean those leafy greens, it's still a must. Have you ever tried looking into one of lettuce heads? It's pretty disturbing that you'd find trapped dust and in some cases, even bugs. You definitely do not want all that to be a part of your green juices. Here are the steps you need to follow for cleaning your leafy greens in the most effective way.

To give your vegetables a *vinegar soak*, fill up a container with cold water and add ½ cup of vinegar into it.

Add your leafy greens into the mixture and make sure that they're completely soaked inside.

Swirl them around. This will help loosen up the dirt and insects that are trapped in the leaves.

Leave them inside for five to ten minutes.

Now, shift them into a colander and rinse them thoroughly with cold water. Make sure you hit every part of your leaves with the water.

Nothing Beats Freshness:

If you're looking to make the most out of your green juicing routines, then freshness is something that you will need to take care of a lot. Veggies are delicate and sensitive beings. Once they're plucked out of their farms, they seem to wilt and dry up really quickly if you're not being careful enough with them.

Apart from affecting their fresh appearance, wilting causes the green juices produced with them to have minimal nutrients and beneficial factors. Who wants that? If you're opting to reject market shelved juices to embrace the true miracles of nature, why not keep the purpose as alive as you can.

It's understandable, that keeping our leafy greens fresh for days is no easy feat. Thankfully, products like *progressive keepers* have gotten you covered on that. They cost as low as ten bucks, and save our veggies that are much more valuable than that.

No More Dodging the Bitterness:

You're going to have to go for the bitter ones, as they are the most effective in keeping you feel healthy. Sure, their grassy and unpleasant isn't something you'd dream of, but you could somewhat stabilize it with a little sweeter fruity additions.

As intimidating as they may taste, the darkest bitter leafy greens are the ones that are the richest in nutrition. Go for more of these, and you'll find yourself feeling a lot better about green juicing as you progress further. Given below are a few benefits worth mentioning, which are specifically achieved through bitter foods.

- They help our bodies to absorb more nutrients from other sources as well, as they digest.

- Our livers get detoxified with their help. This leads to preventing countless diseases.

- They are one of the greatest sources of vitamins and minerals.

- They generally bring down our sugar cravings. This helps in various ways, such as weight loss and prevention from diabetes, etc.

Don't Forget to Switch Up!

As healthy as bitter greens are, there's no reason why you should keep ramming them into your juicer every day. Eating too much of the same thing involves risks too - you never want to keep an identical schedule for the whole week.

Rotating your veggie combos could turn out to be the best way of attaining a wide variety of phytochemicals. A medicine and a poison could be differentiated only on the basis of dosage!

Point is, there's a whole lot of different leafy greens out there, and it's never a good idea to miss out on all but one.

Start Slow – That is Important:

This is an extremely useful tip for people who are looking to start these routines. You must start slow with green juicing – this means that you don't want to give your body crazy doses of detoxifying cleansers right at the start.

Sure, it's a known fact that greens are one of the best things out there for your body, but drinks that are too dense at the start could prove slightly problematic for a beginner. Keep it a bit more dilute in your starting weeks, just to warm your body up for the waves of bitterness it's going to be benefiting from in the near future.

Here's why – a very intense detox could make you feel a bit unsteady and in some cases, even nauseous. This is something you'll have to look out for if you've been a straight-up junk foodie in the past. You must understand your requirements, and work with the suitable ingredients; that's the best way to make the most out of these routines!

The Body's Feedback

You have to listen closely to what your body tells you each day. After crafting and trying out a whole new recipe, pay attention to the feelings you'll experience throughout the day. Ideally, your stomach should feel balanced and remain calm the whole day. That's when you know you can continue adding this drink to your future schedules.

On the other hand, if your stomach churns and growls, leaving you with a queasier feeling; that's a bad sign.

In this case, your body is basically making you aware of the fact that you've consumed something in an intolerable amount, or something you aren't accustomed to digesting.

If your body doesn't seem to accept a specific ingredient, it doesn't mean you have to miss out on its healthful effects completely. The best way to tackle a green juicing problem like this is to start ingesting that ingredient in small amounts, and after regular intervals. This will slowly convince your body that it's fine, you can have it.

However, if you have a complete natural intolerance for something, then that's a whole different scenario. There's no getting used to something like that.

The Perfect Compliment!

This is a very important tip to ensure that you'll be enjoying your drinks instead of chugging them like you're compelled to. Try adding a few healthy sweeteners to cut out the grassy and plain taste of your leafy greens. Apples are the best for this purpose – they help in the proper engagement of gastric enzymes, speeding up the nutrient upload. Feel free to squeeze a lemon into your recipes for that tartness too!

Occasional Juice Cleanses

Juice cleanses are awesome at making you feel a lot fresher and healthier in a matter of just a couple days.

The whole concept is basically giving up on solid foods completely for a short period of time, in order to achieve the following goals:

- Guaranteed weight loss.

- An unmatched boost in energy.

- A much needed detox for the body (especially for the liver).

- Ridding the body of some kind of weakness or disorder.

Juice cleanses, being extremely healthful, should always be made a part of life occasionally by green juicing practitioners. While it's not recommended under certain circumstances to quit ingesting solid food for even a couple of days, it has its own magical benefits.

After all, what sounds wrong about going on a fully nutrient-rich diet for 2-3 days every now and then? It's surely one of the best ways to embrace the most benefits out of the juicing routines.

Doctors Know Best

For all you know, the internet could have information that is not reliable at all. Whatever you find in form of web articles, has no way to be verified besides actually meeting a professional specialist in person. It's best to consult your doctor before designing a green juicing schedule for yourself, as different bodies cater different needs.

The only people who can tell specifically about how **you** can make the most out of your juicing routines, is a doctor who examines your nutrient levels personally. Sure, you can find that general info on the web, but not something that would particularly be suitable for your own body.

With juicing, you're going to be starting a radical transformation phase in your life which must be long term and fun to maintain. This sure does require a professional to watch over what you're taking in, until of course, you become a pro at this yourself. Good luck!

Add These 5 Super Greens to Juice to Fight Against Cancer

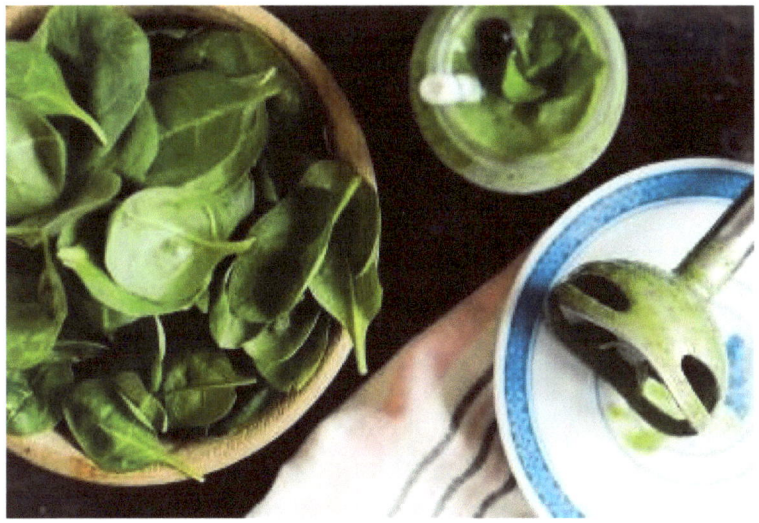

Super greens are known for their innate ability to ward off and fight many different types of medical conditions. One of the most powerful contributions dark greens make toward a healthier you, is their ability to help fight cancer. Many doctors are realizing the importance of incorporating more dark, super greens into a healthy diet for aid in fighting off certain cancers, as well as preventing them from even starting to grow.

Some of the most powerful cancer fighting super greens include:

- **Broccoli**

Broccoli contains a substance known as isothiocyanate that researchers believe sparks genetic changes that are responsible for activating genes that are known to fight cancer while switching off other genes that fuel the tumors. Between the two dynamics, this gives broccoli a huge edge over other vegetables to make it on the list of cancer fighting super greens.

- **Spirulina**

Spirulina is a single-celled algae that has been collected from lakes for thousands of years in multiple parts of the world. A large percentage of Spirulina is made of protein, approximately 60%, and contains many nutrients, including vitamin K and iron. It also contains a high percentage of beta-carotene, more-so than that found in carrots. The blue pigment found in Spirulina has been found to halt the production and spread of cancerous cells, which makes it one of the super greens known to fight cancer and a perfect green to add to your green juice for cancer fighting properties.

- **Bok Choy**

The Chinese cabbage, as it is known, is a neutral, yet slightly sweet green that is full of phytochemical such as thiocyanates, including, indole-3-carbinol, zea-xanthin, isothiocyanates and lutein. All of these are responsible for helping combat such cancers as breast, colon and prostate cancer.

Bok Choy is a powerful super green cancer fighting green that should be added to your green juice on a regular basis.

- **Mustard Greens**

Mustard greens are one of the dark leafy vegetables that are known for being full of a wide range of carotenoids like lutein, saponins, flavonoids and zeaxanthin. These carotenoids act as protectants, according to researchers, to prevent cancer growth in the mouth, larynx and pharynx. It is believed that these carotenoids act like antioxidants by scouring out free radicals in the body and destroying the before they have the ability to become cancerous cells, especially specific types of cancer, such as breast cancer cells, lung cancer, stomach cancer and skin cancer cells. When you add mustard greens to your green juice on a daily basis, you are feeding your body powerful anti-cancer fighting agents for a fighting chance.

- **Collard Greens**

Collard greens are one of the highest contenders of greens for vitamin C and excellent source of vitamin K along with soluble fiber. Although this is all good news, the best news comes from the cancer fighting properties known as sulforphane and diindolymethane. Collards have a unique distinction among greens in that they are rich in sulfa-containing compounds. Glucosinolates support detoxification while indole-3-carbinol works to reduce the risk of lung, breast and colon cancers. Juice collard greens in your green juice daily to help prevent and fight cancer.

Final Thoughts

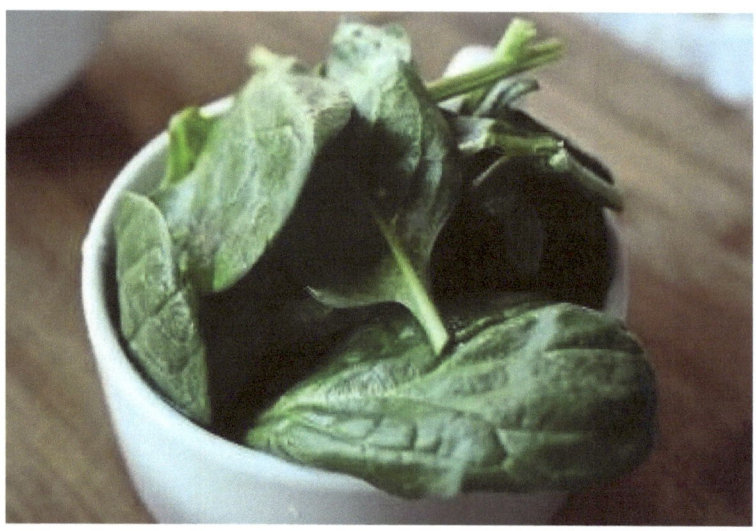

It's no secret. The benefits of green juicing are well documented, and the list of people whose health has been completely transformed by the nutritionally-loaded super juice just keeps on growing. But if you need more inspiration before making green juicing part of your daily dietary regimen, consider this important statement: A green juice a day keeps the doctor away.

Sounds too good to be true, you say? Mere words that lack medical evidence and the backing of scientific research? If you are skeptical that green juicing can be the gateway into the vibrant and healthy lifestyle of which you have always dreamed, you may want to think again. The truth is that green juicing can indeed significantly reduce your trips to the doctor's office.

Now before you dismiss this article as the hyped up language of a medical quack pedaling the latest cure-all remedy, let me voice agreement that bold claims must stand up under scrutiny and need to be based in the realm of reality. There simply must be some significant evidence that green drinks really can transform human health if the claim is to be believed.

So based on this understanding, here are two of the most compelling reasons that green juice stands out as an amazing nutritional powerhouse that can literally transform and rejuvenate the body while reducing one's frequency of illness and need for medical intervention:

1) **Green juice directly nourishes the body at the cellular level:** Think back to high school biology class. What did the teacher tell your class about the cell? It is the basic unit of structure and function in living things. This very important fact provides insight into a basic truth about human health. Simply stated, the body maintains proper health if the cells are properly nourished.

So the key to good health is to nourish the trillions of cells in the human body as directly and efficiently as possible. Here is where the magnificent value of green juice comes into play. All of the vitamins and nutrients packed in the green juice drink are released into the body in liquid form, allowing for faster absorption by body systems and having a more direct impact on body cells than solid foods that require the process of digestion before nutrients can be absorbed.

2) **Green juice contains chlorophyll:** Think back again to the biology classroom. The chlorophyll in green plants is an amazing substance that allows them to use sunlight to create chemical energy. Ingested by humans, chlorophyll has a cleansing and detoxifying effect on the lymph system, blood, cells, organ systems, and glands of the body. This removes disease causing wastes that can build up in the body over time.

In addition, chlorophyll taken into the body through green foods is known to provide the following benefits:

- stabilizing of blood sugar

- maintaining of high red blood cell count

- promotion of better blood circulation

- reduction of inflammation

- cleansing of bowels

- removal of toxins from specific organs such as the liver.

Green foods that contain chlorophyll include barley grass, wheat grass, kale, spinach, alfalfa, mustard greens, cabbage, and asparagus. When these greens are juiced, they compose a nutritionally and chlorophyll dense drink capable of completely revitalizing the body.

Given the amazing benefits of green juice, it is no surprise that it is often referred to as a 'superfood'. Get started today with green juicing, and discover for yourself that a green juice a day keeps the doctor away!

Omega Juicers VRT350X

The Omega Juicer VRT350X (http://amzn.to/2cFDoSD) is a great juicer for either fine or coarse juicing. This juicer will process vegetables or fruit. It also juices wheat grass which is a very nutritious plant. The low speed juicing system installed in the Omega Juicer VRT350X enables you to get more nutrients out of what you are juicing without as much waste.

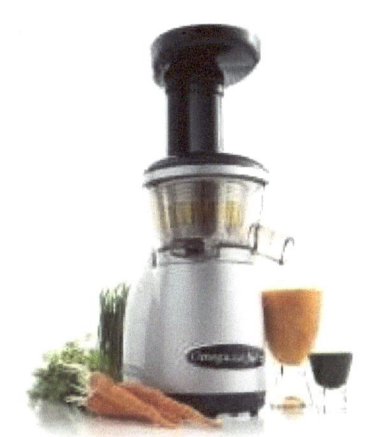

Some people are partial to a lot of pulp in their juice while others prefer a less pulpy mixture. This juicer makes it possible to choose how much pulp you actually want in your juice. The way this is made possible is through the fine and coarse juicing screens. Automatic pulp ejection is what enables this juicer to juice wheat grass, some juicers are unable to juice this plant.

The Omega Juicer VRT350X is also very compact and only weighs 17.7 pounds. One of the main features that I find attractive is the auto cleaning system. Some juicers have to be cleaned of pulp in between each load of fruits and vegetables otherwise the screen gets clogged up and you do not have as much of a juice production.

With the auto cleaning system the screen is kept as clear as possible to allow more juice to come out. You do have to clean the juicer once you are done using it but having the auto cleaning function can make the job easier and take a lot less time.

Unlike other juicers the Omega Juicers VRT350X is very quiet while juicing so there is less loud noise that you have to deal with. I have had a juicer in the past, the noise it made and the clean up afterwards were the two worst things. So, I was thrilled when I read about all the Omega Juicers VRT350X had to offer.

Juicing fruits and vegetables is much healthier than getting store bought juice, less sugars and preservatives. Choosing a juicer can be hard though however, with the Omega Juicers VRT350X you are getting a great quality juicer for a good price of $204.00. If you buy through my link above, I'll get a small commission.

You can find other Omega models and other brands by doing a search on Amazon for "juicers".

Other Juicing Books by This Author

If you would like to read more about juicing, here is a list of the titles, CreateSpace links and descriptions:

Fight Cancer With Juicing
https://www.createspace.com/6155567

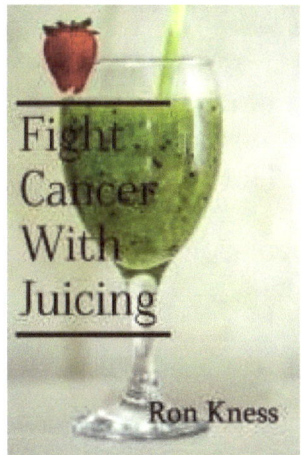

Juicing is a healthy practice that has allowed millions of people to boost their nutrition. Juicing fruits and vegetables provides you important antioxidants, which scavenge for oxygen free radicals that can damage cellular structures, including DNA. When DNA is damaged, it can result in mutations that lead to cancer.

Well-balanced nutrition from a variety of healthy whole foods helps support and maintain on-going good health, and experts agree that nutrition plays a key role in preventing chronic and terminal illness.

When juicing is done right, that is when the majority of your juice blends is comprised of vegetables and very low sugar fruit, you can easily boost your nutritional intake thereby improving your health and lower your risks for cancer.

This book gives you the information needed to not only help prevent cancer in the first place, but to help fight it naturally if you already have it.

Juicing for Health: The Complete Guide to Juicing for Good Nutrition

https://www.createspace.com/6241849

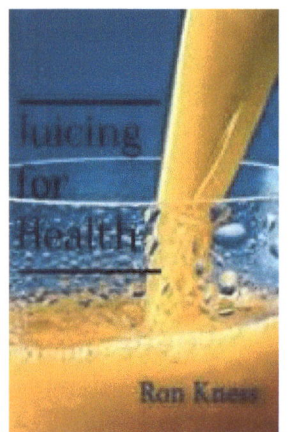

It's well documented that many of us need to increase our daily intake of fruit and vegetables. We are the champions of the world when it comes to getting enough of the macronutrients carbs, protein, and fat, but we're sorely lacking when it comes to getting more micronutrients.

While the Centers For Disease Control recommend adults consume about 1 ½ to 2 cups of fruit and 2 to 3 cups of vegetables daily, an analysis of American diets between 2007 and 2010 found that 50% of the population ate less than 1 cup of fruit and less than 1 ½ cups of vegetables.

An astounding 76% of people did not eat nearly enough fruit, and 87% did not eat enough vegetables.

Many people simply don't like eating vegetables. Broccoli is tough, cabbage is chewy, and carrots can break your teeth if they haven't been boiled long enough and let's not get started on that stringy asparagus!

However, fruit and vegetables are where essential micronutrients are to be found and juicing is a great way to easily pack more of them into a well-balanced and healthy diet.

Thousands have joined the juicing revolution and for good reason, it is healthy, convenient and allows you to get key vitamins and minerals from plant foods that may be missing from your diet.

Juicing Your Way to Better Health

https://www.createspace.com/6558396

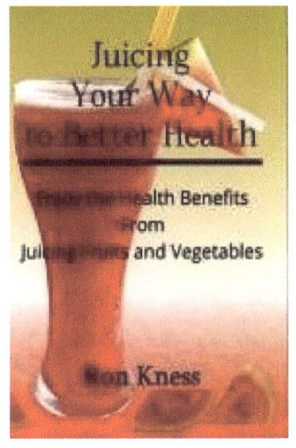

Whether it is just a fad or a trend that is here to stay, juicing is extremely popular among health conscious individuals. As more and more people experience the amazing results associated with this healthy lifestyle choice, its popularity is expected to grow.

Without question, juicing can be incorporated into your daily life to increase your overall health and vitality. By increasing your daily intake of healthy fruits and vegetables, you'll be giving your body the essential building blocks it needs. To get the most benefit out of juicing, you'll want to educate yourself on some of the basics before you get started. In my book "Juicing Your Way to Better Health", you'll find a wealth of information on juicing.

If you are new to juicing, you may find the process to be a bit of a hassle. However, once you start to see and experience the many benefits associated with juicing, you may wonder how you ever got along without it. So commit to testing out your new lifestyle using juice from fruits and vegetables for at least several weeks before deciding if it is for you or not.

About the Author

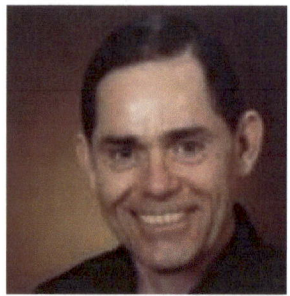

I grew up in Central Minnesota, where my parents owned and operated a fishing resort. Once out of high school I tried a couple of semesters of college, only to quit halfway through the Spring term; I decided at that time that college wasn't for me.

Then I decided to follow my father's previous occupation as an auto mechanic. I graduated from a two-year of vocational training course and worked as a mechanic for five years. While in vocational training, I decided to join the National Guard where I eventually ended up working full-time for 32 years.

So how does all of this relate to writing? In one of my leadership schools, the instructor, who was an English teacher at a juvenile detention center, presented writing to me in a whole new way - a way that started to develop my interest in working with words.

I eventually went back to college on the GI Bill while I was working and earned my Bachelor's degree in Business Administration. Taking a class or two per semester at night and on weekends took me seven years to complete my degree.

Fast forward about 40 years and I now have published over 75 books on Amazon for Kindle, CreateSpace and other publishing platforms.

Besides my own writing, I also ghostwrite ebooks, reports, articles, blogs and do Kindle conversions for clients on a variety of topics.

Today my wife and I are retired from our careers and live in Gold Canyon, AZ. I now write as a retirement business where you'll find me happily sitting in my office typing away on my laptop as I work on my next book or ghostwriting project . . . that is if we are not traveling on a cruise ship - our new-found mode of travel.